MENTAL HEALTH CARE FOR THE ELDERLY

How They Respond Differently From Young People

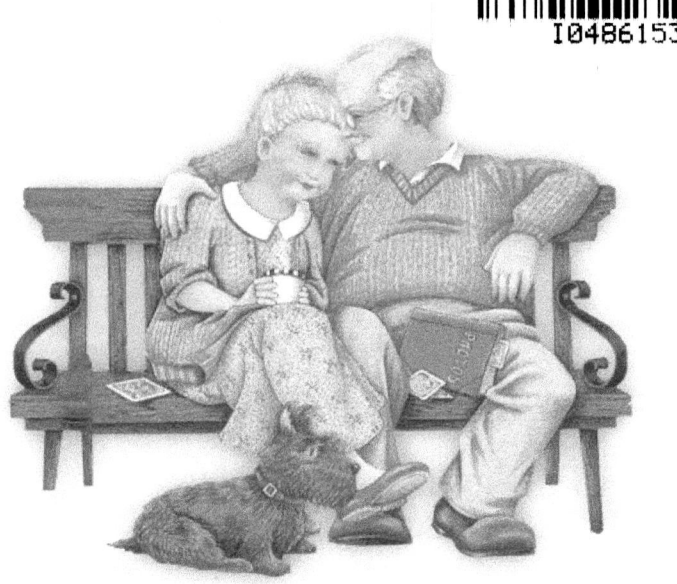

By Patricia A Carlisle

Introduction

I want to thank you and congratulate you for choosing the book, *"MENTAL HEALTH CARE FOR THE ELDERLY: How They Respond Differently from Young People"*.

All over the world the ageing population increases on a regular basis. The elderly accounts for the populations in the age group from sixty years and above. In most countries, these age groups are either referred to as dependants, those within the retirement age, or they are commonly referred to as the aged.

Hence, mental health care for the elderly is a topic that needs to be taken seriously, because we have often witnessed the emotional problems associated with the well being of these adults, and it is very important that they be taken into high consideration at this time of their lives.

Thanks again for choosing this book, I hope you enjoy it!

TABLE OF CONTENT

STRATEGIES IN MENTAL HEALTH CARE

Conclusion

Preview Of 'HOW TO LIVE WITH PEOPLE AFFECT WITH MENTAL ILLNESS'

Bonus: Subscribe To The FREE BOOK

Chapter 1

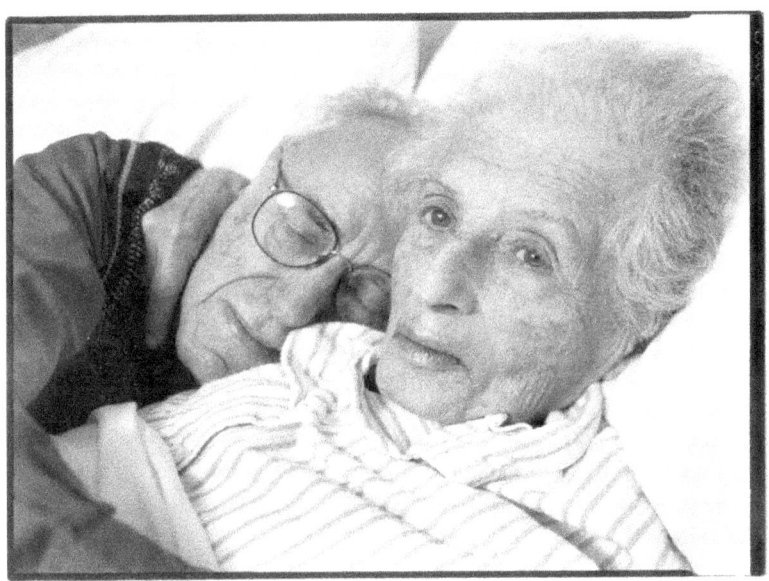

ELDERLY POPULATION

The population of the elderly though, is not uniform around the world. For instance, countries with higher life expectancy rate like China, have more numbers of the elderly in its population than any other country. This is largely due to the care given to the elderly, and the high level of activities that tends to cause low level of mortality rates among the elderly, activities like spiritual exercises, yoga, natural medicinal herbs and roots intake, which is what helps to maintain balance and healthy body cells. This is a tradition in China that has led to their life expectancy to be higher.

Elderly people are highly appreciated for their immense contribution to society. The fact that they are members of the family, and they play advisor roles in families helps the effects of aging. They are not necessarily part of the workforce, or more often their working activities is reduced drastically due to aging, the elderly that still engage in active service tend to develop mental disorders, and some other health problems like neurological problems, hearing loss, addiction to substance used for treatments of other health issues associated with ageing, diabetes, and osteoarthritis. The problem of encountering several other health problems tends to appear in the long run. The World Health Organization reported that about 15 percent of the elderly above 60 years of age generally develop mental disorders.

Chapter 2

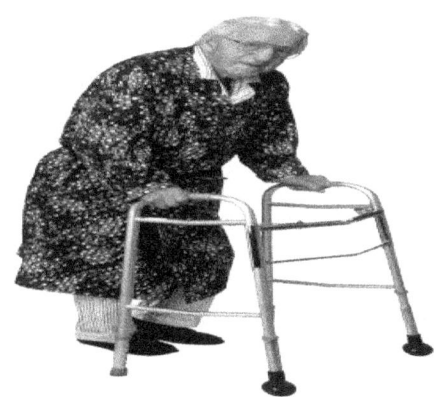

PROBLEMS ASSOCIATED WITH THE ELDERLY

It might interest you to know that there are certain problems associated with the mental abilities of the elderly. Some of the problems experienced by the elderly are the Neuropsychiatric disorders which are common among them. The Neuropsychiatric disorders accounts for about 7 percent of the complete incapacities of the elderly. The elderly occasionally have this inability to remember a lot of things that they need to do, and this often lead to them always needing someone to assist them in different capacity. They cannot act alone, or they find it very difficult to live alone without having someone around them.

The elderly that suffers from neuropsychiatric disorders often require their grand children to visit them frequently during holidays, and they really love to have their grand children around them. But young people do not have the same mentality, the young people like to be with their peer groups or friends, most often will spend their time playing games, going to clubs, or chasing their dreams or career.

Chapter 3

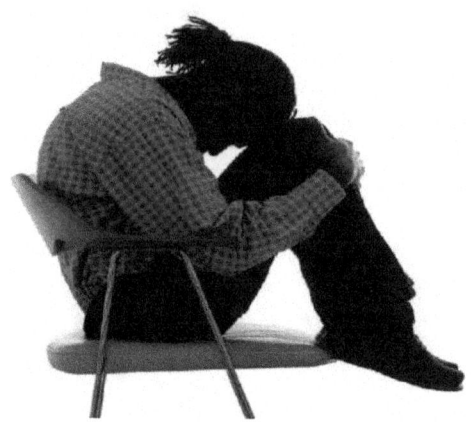

MENTAL HEALTH CARE FOR YOUNG PEOPLE

Now talking about the mental health care for the elderly, and how they respond differently from the young people. After having said that, we ask the question if there is a need for mental health care for young adults. You might wonder why? We also know that young people sometimes fall victims to so many societal vices, and to solve the puzzle we consider the circumstances where there might be a need for mental care.

Every young person needs mental care from the cradle, a young person needs to grow and develop in a favorable environment where he or she will actually conform to the expected "norms" in society. If these factors are missing or limited, they will definitely be a problem when the child or young person does not develop properly, and fit in the society "norm". All over the world, there are instances and places where young people are considered as societal misfit, and are contributing to the problems of the world. Today there are millions of young people who are lured into drug abuse.

These youngsters start to use drugs, and destroy their lives and many times become a nuisance in society, and cause a lot of problems. They get caught in criminal activities, and sometimes become victims of crimes as well. The females are sometimes lured into sexual activities; drug trafficking, child trafficking, and so many other societal vices which often times cause them to live a wasteful life, and serve long jail terms.

Chapter 4

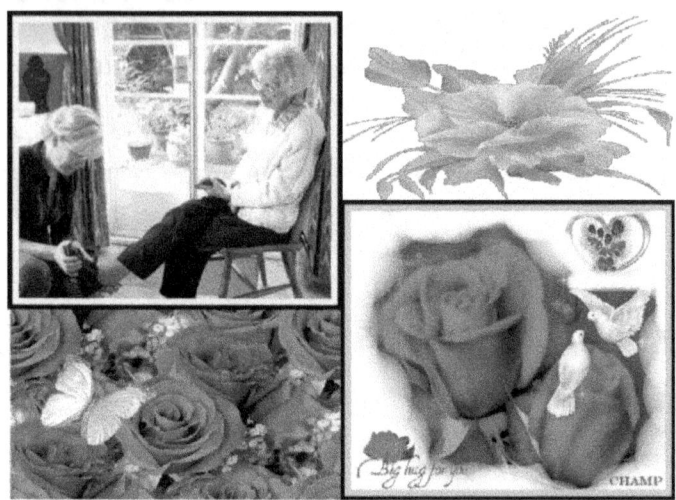

MENTAL CARE FOR THE ELDERLY AND YOUNG ADULTS

Mental care needed by young adults is completely different from that of the elderly. The elderly are more connected to their well being, and there are factors which they continue to fight against and suppress. It's a common feature that the elderly are more prone to weakness. Their physical fitness comes into test, and their strength often lets them down, this contributes largely to the mental stress and unhealthiness when they continuously think that they are being left out or ostracized.

While young people really need help in terms of their steady mental development, when they encounter problems such as those that were mention earlier, they sometimes do not bring it to the awareness of their parents, only a few are able to do so, and only vigilant parents are able to understand the problems the young person is facing outside the home. That is why parents need to maintain good communication with their children at all times, and must not give room for laxity in that regard.

The response to mental health care by young adults can be very irrational; making a young person get the mental health needed for further development can be misinterpreted, and mean a different thing entirely than the understanding of the elderly. Some people may see a problem having to make efforts to trust the information he or she is receiving. When there is a rule, or strict adherence to be followed a young person will understand that it is for his or her own benefit at least for today's subject, he or she may have a problem of following strict rules.

Chapter 5

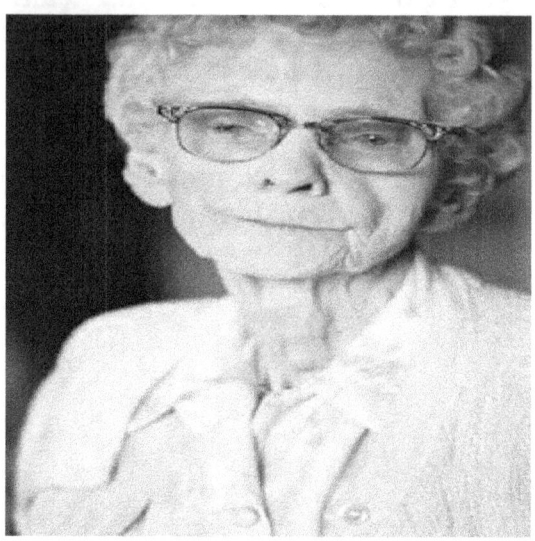

INSIGHT OF ELDERLY MENTAL HEALTH CARE

The insight of the elderly towards mental health care is easily determinable, the elderly has more experience in life, and knows exactly what he or she wants, how he or she is feeling, and what is really disturbing to them. And as such, they are more capable of being approached, and given the necessary treatment they desire. Some however, may be irrational, but elderly individuals often have the insight that there is something that is worthy in mental health care, the elderly realizes that he or she is aging, and probably will need all the necessary medical attention that they require, and are more likely to cooperate and experience a successful outcome.

The elderly are more attentive to details and outcome of their mental health issues concerning their wellbeing. The majority of the elderly at that stage of life are incline to living a good life free of stress, but what they are facing can sometimes be the direct opposite when health challenges begin to develop. While the health issues of the young may be different from that of the elderly, their responses are totally different depending on the issues involved. Health challenges of the elderly are definitely different, issues such as heart attacks, stroke, obesity, arthritis, body pains, senility etc.- while that of the young may be something that deals with growing up, physical and mental development, intellectual and educationally learning problems. It could also range from skin, disease related issues which can affect mental health of the young, they do not experience at that stage in life the same level of mental health challenges posed to the elderly

Chapter 6

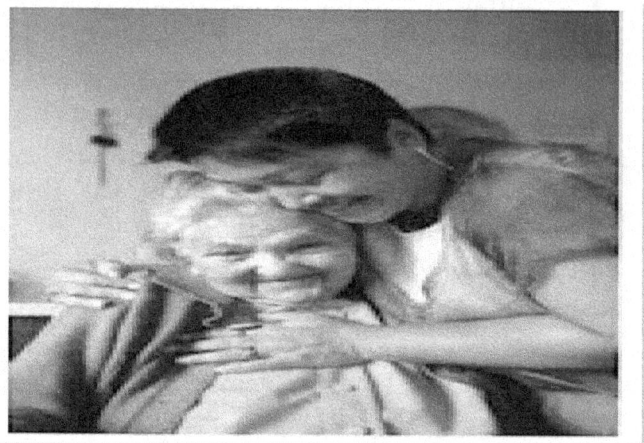

PSYCHOLOGICAL AND OTHER FORMS OF SYMPTOMS IN YOUNG OR OLD

As life continues, stress factors begin to appear for the elderly, although stress is generally a common phenomenon to all people, most elderly people tend to lose touch of their abilities to exist independently because their mobility tend to be limited. Now we can see that this is a major factor. While this is different for a young person who still has the energy to move around. Like it was discussed earlier on, frailty is a major problem that forms in the elderly. Also, they may experience a decline in mental or physical disposition which would make them really need long term mental health care.

The elderly often lose their love ones easily, and because of deaths that occur to their partners, this might take a longer time to get over, and this may cause a big problem for the partner that is left behind, the response to this kind of situation can make them feel very depressed, and this may cause some mental health challenges to the elderly, but the younger person's responses maybe quite different entirely since they are still young and they are able to move on in life.

SOCIAL LIFE: The quality of your social life can have a big effect on you mental health. Age causes some elderly individuals to reduce, or have little or no social life, and this tends to affect their social economic status. Events such as retirement or disability may drastically affect the lifestyle of the elderly. But in the young person these late life activities does not hinder their social life, since they are not involve in retirement, or there is no need for economic change in their situation.

It is rarely seen for the young person to suffer isolation, because they always have their peer group to get involve with, they rarely have this type of loneliness, depression, or any psychological distress as experienced by the elderly. Responses to mental health has an impact on the physical health of older people, the conditions of their health such as hearing loss, are common among the elderly, more depression are occurring in high rates in elderly who have medical issues. It is also to be noted that many times the non treatment of health issues such as heart diseases, can adversely affect the result of the physical well being of the elderly, and also give rise to other disease related to such conditions.

Chapter 7

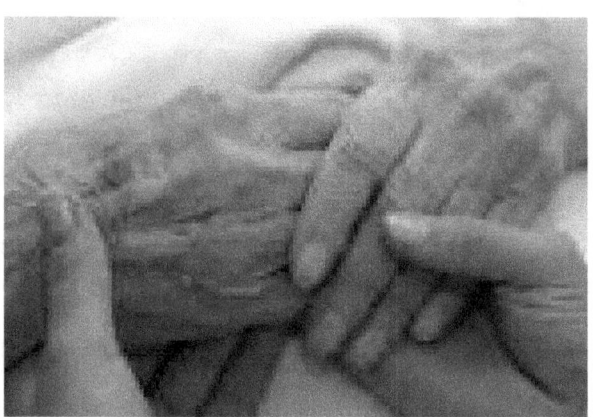

HOW ELDERLY RESPOND TO MENTAL HEALTH PROBLEMS

The elderly are vulnerable to elder abuses- there are cases of physical assault, sexual abuse, emotional, material, financial, and psychological abuse of the elderly by others who are living, leaving them with the feeling of being ignored, neglected, and abused with disrespect for their dignity.

The abuse of the elders can lead not only to physical injuries, but also litigations and this affects the mental health of the elderly, and how they respond to this will be very different from the way the younger person will respond. The elderly person or family member may press charges to enforce his or her rights when they become aware. While the younger person may know little, or what to do when faced with similar incidence at any point in time. The outcome of these challenges posed by these types of threats is the consequences of depression, anxiety and long lasting psychological problems for the elders.

The elderly are prone to mental health problems like Dementia and depression, and this is a growing mental health concerns. The syndrome although not a normal constituent of aging, causes deterioration in memory, changes in behavior, thinking and reduction in the ability to carry out day to day activities. The effects of these syndromes on the older people are quite large. The responses to this kind of mental health care for them can be quite challenging, many times they seem to feel very sorry for themselves, and almost hoping that their time is up for them. Medical practitioners always find it hard trying to convince them to stay positive about their health, and that their health can always improve.

Chapter 8

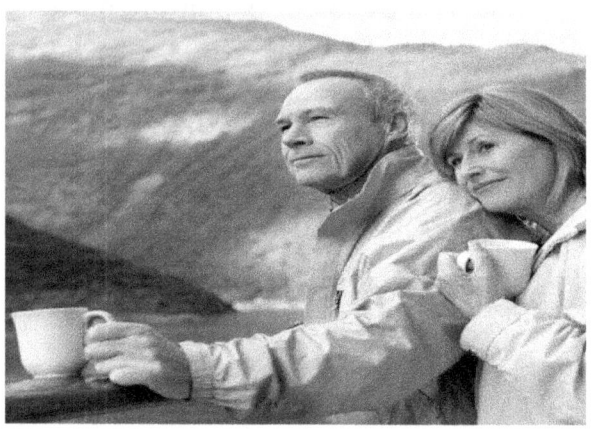

MENTAL HEALTH CHALLENGES

For the young adults who are undergoing rehabilitation due to drug abuse which has affected his or her mental well being, the reaction is different. Considering the effects and influence that drugs have caused on a younger persons mental well being can actually caused an imbalance in their level of thinking. The rehabilitation process may be hindered by chronic effect of the drugs to the extent that the mental health care may be stretch to its limit. When their numbers increase it causes a societal problem considering the huge funds, medical personnel, and services that will be needed to contain the resultant effect.

MENTAL HEALTH CARE FOR THE ELDERLY

While mental care for the elders does not pose a threat, that of the younger persons undergoing mental rehabilitations can be threatening to not only the medical personnel's in charge, but also a menace to the society at large. Hence, the response of both the younger persons and the elderly to mental health care in this aspect is very different.

The elderly do not need to be forced to receive mental health care; in fact they see it as something that is good for their well being and good health. Many elderly people accept the fact they need the mental health care services when it is a facility provided by the government. The young person's responses (if it is in response to mental cases), are different because it has to do with some level of control. The younger person is energetic; the need for forcing them to receive the treatment will always arise at some point.

For the young person "mental health care" may be scary, the temptation to skip treatment may arise, he or she might not realize the benefits, or they need to receive mental care treatment. The young age may not help matters when they become opposed to mental health treatment. The series of process that they might need to go through to establish, or complete the mental health care treatment sometimes can make them become skeptical, or avoid receiving treatment, these scenarios paints the true pictures of responses of both the elderly and young when it comes to mental health.

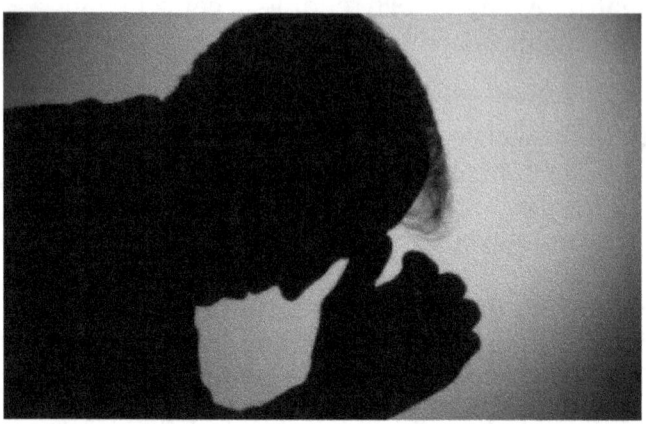

Chapter 9

DEPRESSION AND THE ELDERLY

As elderly people suffer more mental depression than younger people the efforts required to create awareness and treatments are always there in the health sector, but the response to receive treatment is not a priority for the young person.

Elderly people are quicker to respond to mental health checks than younger individuals. Probably the younger individuals feel less concerned, and think he or she is unconnected with this care. A young adult is more likely to visit a psychotherapy more often than the elderly.

While the elders always lay emphasis on their life experiences in response to visiting a therapist, the younger person's conception is based on curiosity, and the need to determine whether the situation is worth visiting a therapist or not.

Chapter 10

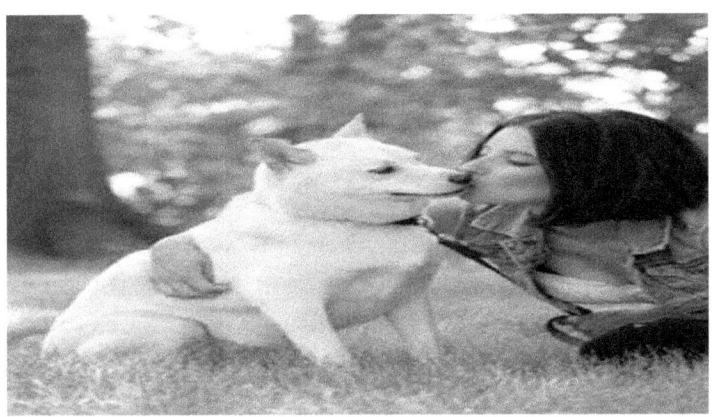

STRATEGIES IN MENTAL HEALTH CARE

 The strategy employed in mental health care consist of a series of training for professional health workers, ways of preventing, and managing diseases associated with the elderly which includes neurological, mental and substance uses disorders, drawing out a sustainable plan, and long term strategy to care for the elderly and the young, and an friendly environment that will justify quality service delivery, in that way we can be able to monitor and understand the various reasons of both the elderly and the young in responses to mental health care delivery. This will also enable the government to determine the necessary approach to mental health care deliveries.

Also, promoting mental health care for older people will improve active and healthy aging, when the young adults are given their retirement age, and the benefits of getting quality health services, this will also prompt them to put in more hard work in their various lives endeavors to maximize productivity. Creating an environment with good conditions and lifestyle that support good health will play a big role in how the elderly and the young will react to health care.

Conclusion

Thank you again for choosing this book!

In order to bring together both parties to accept and agree with the quality of mental health care so there will be no differentiation in responses, the Government should create the best enabling environment that will support both the old and the young to respond the same way, and not differently.

For instance, providing security and liberty; enough housing via supportive housing policy, supporting the social lives of the populations of the elderly, social and health programs channeled towards the vulnerable categories of members of the public, like those who live in solitude, the rural populace, or even those who suffer mental or chronic physical illness.

Providing programs that; will eradicate and deal with abuse of the elderly in the society, and also providing community development programs. These are some of the ways that will influence how both the elderly and the young will respond to mental health care positively and move in the right direction.

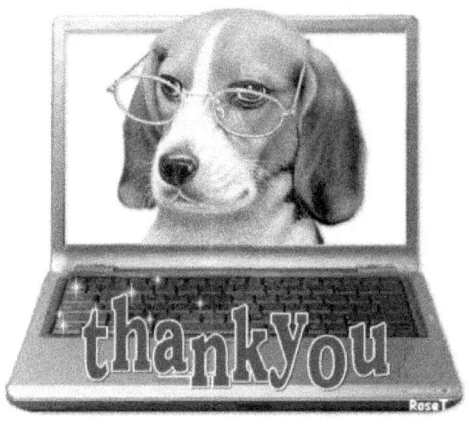

Finally, if you enjoyed this book, would you be kind enough to leave a review for this book on Amazon? It'd be greatly appreciated!

Thank you and good luck!

Preview Of 'HOW TO LIVE WITH PEOPLE AFFECT WITH MENTAL ILLNESS'

Chapter 1

INTRODUCTION

Stigma associated with mental illness and psychiatric treatment, and the discrimination towards people with mental illnesses that frequently results from this, are the main obstacles preventing early and successful treatment. To reduce such stigma and discrimination towards mentally ill people and especially those with schizophrenia, the World Psychiatric Association's (WPA) anti stigma programmed 'Open the Doors' is currently being implemented in more than 20 countries. The programmed has been undertaken in seven project centers in Germany. Public information programs and education measures aimed at selected target groups are intended to improve the public's knowledge regarding symptomatolgy, causes and treatment options for schizophrenia. Improved knowledge should in turn reduce prejudice and negative education. Protest and contact are the key elements of anti stigma strategies recommended by the WPA and various research groups.

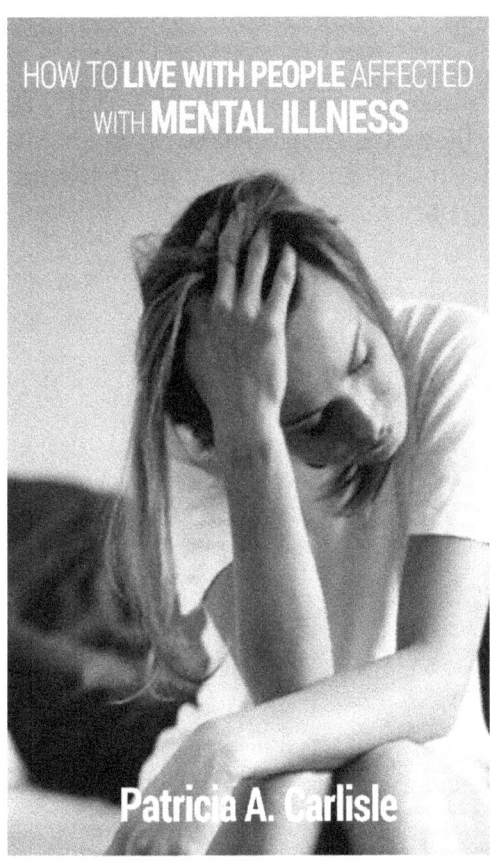

HOW TO **LIVE WITH PEOPLE** AFFECTED WITH **MENTAL ILLNESS**

Patricia A. Carlisle

How to live with people affected with mental illness.

Check Out My Other Books

Below you'll find some of my other popular books that are popular on Amazon and Kindle as well. Alternatively, you can visit my author page on Amazon to see other work done by me. (https://amazon.com/author/patriciacarlisle)

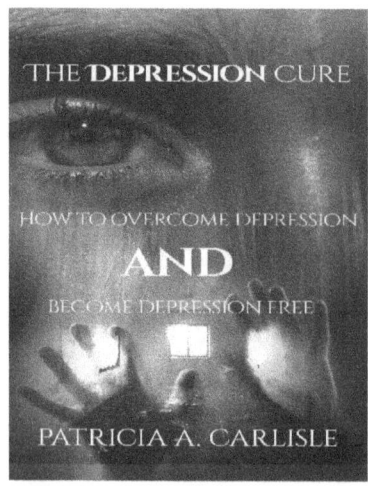

THE DEPRESSION CURE: How to overcome depression and become depression free.

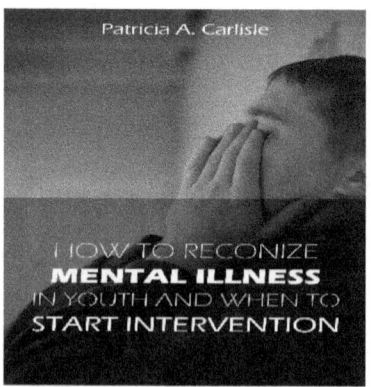

HOW TO RECOGNIZE MENTAL ILLNESS IN YOUTH: and When to Start Intervention:

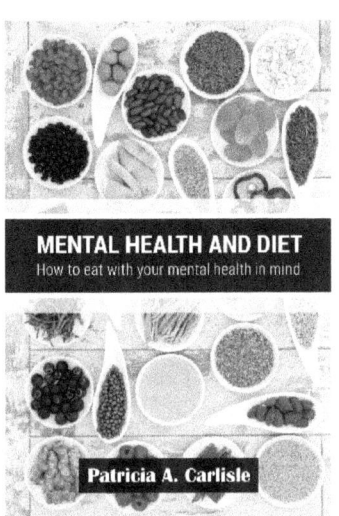

Mental Health and diet: How to eat with your mental health in mind.

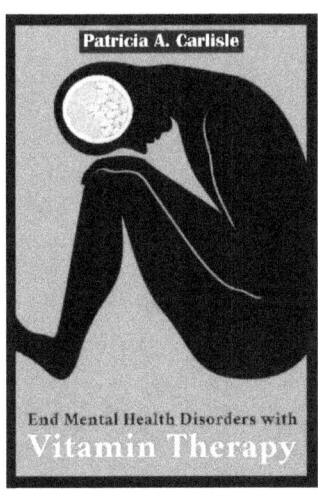

End Mental Disorders with vitamin therapy.

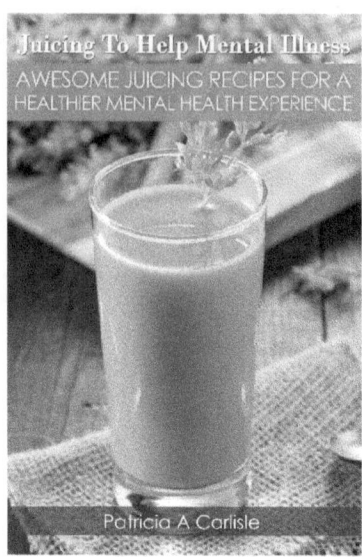

Juicing to Help Mental Illness: Awesome juicing recipes for a healthier mental health.

You can simply search for these titles on the Amazon website to find them.

BONUS: SUBSCRIBE TO THE FREE BOOK

Beginners Guide to Yoga & Meditation

"Stressed out? Do You Feel Like The World Is Crashing Down Around You? Want To Take A Vacation That Will Relax Your Mind, Body And Spirit? Well this Easy To Read Step By Step

E-Book Makes It All Possible!"

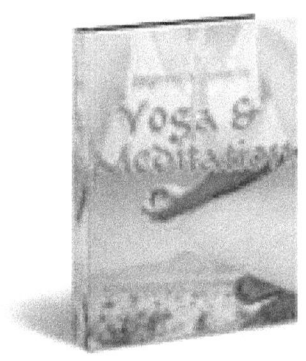

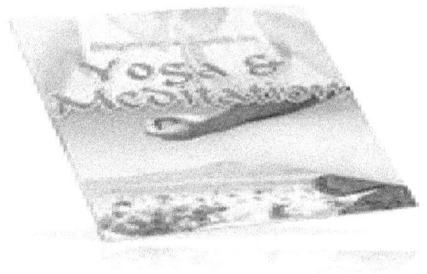

Instructions on how to join our mailing list, and receive a free copy of "Yoga and Meditation" can be found in any of my Kindle eBooks.

NOTES

NOTES

NOTES

NOTES

www.ingramcontent.com/pod-product-compliance
Lightning Source LLC
Chambersburg PA
CBHW070750180526
45168CB00004B/1577